Intermittent Fasting

A Scientifically Proven Approach to Intermittent Fasting and Ketogenic Diet. Fasting Plan and Schedule, Benefits, Tips and Success Stories - Start Burning More Calories While You Sleep!

by Lee Strong

INTRODUCTION	1
CHAPTER 1 WHAT IS INTERMITTENT FASTING?	3
CHAPTER 2 THE PHYSIOLOGY OF FASTING	5
CHAPTER 3 WHY FAST?	9
CHAPTER 4 BUSTING MYTHS AND MISCONCEPTIONS OF FASTING	19
CHAPTER 5 CHOOSE YOUR FASTING PLAN	23
CHAPTER 6 GET STARTED AS A BEGINNER	26
CHAPTER 7 AVOIDING COMMON FASTING MISTAKES	31
CHAPTER 8 INTERMITTENT FASTING AND THE KETOGENIC DIET	34
CHAPTER 9 INTERMITTENT FASTING FOR WOMEN	37
CHAPTER 10 FASTING TIPS TO MAKE THE FAST WORK FOR YOU	41
CHAPTER 11 Q & A	48
CHAPTER 12 SUCCESS STORIES WITH INTERMITTENT FASTING	55
CONCLUSION	57

☐ **Copyright 2019 by Self-Publishing Mastery - All rights reserved**

No part of this publication may be reproduced or transmitted in say form or by any means, mechanical or electronic including photocopying and recording, or by any information storage and retrieval systems without permission in writing from author or publisher (except by reviewer, who may quote brief passages and/or show brief video clips in a review.)

The information provided herein is stated to be truthful and consistent, in that any liability, in terms of inattention or otherwise, by any usage or abuse of any policies, processes, or directions contained within is the solitary and utter responsibility of the recipient reader. Under no circumstances will any legal responsibility or blame be held against the publisher for any reparation, damages or momentary loss due to the information herein, either directly or indirectly.

You must not rely on the information in this book as an alternative to medical advice from your doctor or other professional healthcare providers.

If you have any specific questions about any medical matter you should consult your doctor or other professional healthcare providers.

You should never delay seeking medical advice, disregard medical advice, or discontinue medical treatment because of information in this book.

Introduction

Intermittent fasting is the easiest thing you can do for guaranteed weight loss and health benefits. Intermittent fasting is a lifestyle that many people have started to adopt recently. Many confuse this eating pattern with a diet. Intermittent fasting is not a diet, rather a lifestyle change. It is a revolutionary weightless system to shrink fat cells, boost your metabolism, and improve the quality of your life.

Humans are designed to eat good foods and fast for a period of time. This is the reason why fasting has been practiced since ancient times. The problem is that in recent times, we get caught up in eating too much junk food too often. This comprehensive guide delivers you a guaranteed weight loss plan. Intermittent fasting is not all about weight loss. Studies show that this eating plan has powerful effects on your body and brain.

It can decrease your appetite, lowers your risk of heart disease, minimize your risk of type-2 diabetes, detoxify your body of harmful toxins, and increase longevity. No more excuses, no more masking over the problem, it's time to transform your life forever.

If you have been looking for a healthy eating plan to suit your lifestyle that will help you lose weight and stay in shape, then this Intermittent Fasting guide is for you!

Get Your Copy Today!

Chapter 1: What is Intermittent Fasting?

The concept of intermittent fasting is not new. Intermittent fasting is the process of avoiding food and calorie-rich drinks for a certain amount of time. Intermittent fasting or IF involves a cycle of eating and fasting. It is an eating pattern where one shift to periods of eating and fasting over a given period of time. There is nothing set in stone about it and you can do different types of intermittent fasting. Intermittent fasting isn't a diet. It is a way of eating that humans have been doing for centuries.

Don't confuse starvation with fasting. Fasting is completely different from starvation in one crucial way: control. Starvation is the involuntary abstention from eating. Fasting, on the other hand, is voluntary abstention from eating for health, weight loss, spiritual or other reasons. Food is readily available, but you choose not to eat it. Fasting has no standard duration. Anytime you are not eating and skipping meals are technically fasting. For example, you may fast between dinner and breakfast the next day. It will be 12 hours fast.

History of fasting

From an evolutionary standpoint, a modern eating habit of eating three meals a day and snacking throughout the day is not ideal for survival or good health. Before the agricultural invitation, food availability was unpredictable and highly irregular. War, drought, disease and insect infestations, all played a part in restricting food; something triggered starvation. Periods without food could last weeks or even months.

As human societies developed agriculture, these famines and famine type situations gradually reduced. However, ancient civilizations, like the Egyptian, and the Greeks, recognized there was something deeply intrinsically beneficial to periodic fasting. As famine eliminated, ancient cultures replaced them with periods of voluntary fasting. Fasting was often called time of "purification," "detoxification," and "cleansing." Ancient Greek records show an unyielding belief in the power of fasting. Fasting is the most time-honored and widespread healing tradition in the world.

The early advocates

Hippocrates of Cos (c. 460–c. 370 BC), was one of the early fasting advocates. He is considered as the father of modern medicine. Obesity was a problem during his time. Hippocrates mentioned, "Sudden death is more common in obese people than learn." His recommendation was that obese people should eat only once during the day. Meaning he prescribed a 24-hour fast for obese people. He also recommends physical exercise and a high-fat diet.

The ancient Greek writer and historian Plutarch (c. 46–c. 120) agreed with Hippocrates. He wrote, "It is better to fast, instead of using medicine." Renowned ancient Greek thinkers Plato and his student Aristotle were also staunch supporters of fasting.

The ancient Greeks believed that fasting to be a natural remedy for illness. The ancient Greeks also believed that fasting improved mental and cognitive abilities. Even one of America's founding fathers, Benjamin Franklin (1706–1790) wrote, "the best of all medicines is resting and fasting."

Besides the health benefits, people are fasting for a religious region for centuries. Buddhism, Judaism, Christianity, Hinduism, and Islam, all incorporate fasting in ritual practice. Fasting is even mentioned in the Bible. Matthew 4:2 states, "Then Jesus was led by the Spirit into the wilderness to be tempted by the devil. After fasting forty days and forty nights, he was hungry."

Chapter 2: The Physiology of Fasting

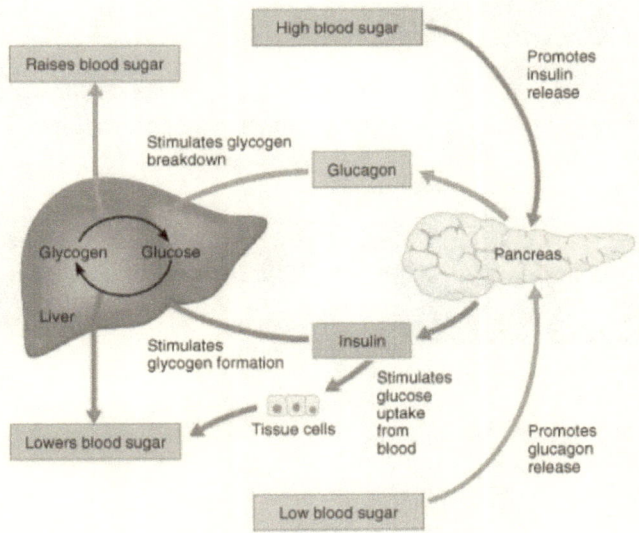

    Intermittent fasting is a way of eating and not eating. You restrict your food consumption for a certain time frame. The human body exists generally in two states, fed and fasted. Fed state is after you have eaten, digesting and are now circulating the blood system. The fasted stage happens when all of the fuel (glucose) has run out. It happens if you fast for 7 to 8 hours. These two the states are different sides of the same coin. Either your body is storing calories or burning calories.

Intermittent Fasting States

Fed State
- Starts when you begin eating
- Lasts for 3 to 5 hours

Post-Absorptive State
- Your body isn't processing a meal
- Lasts until 8 to 12 hours after your last meal

Fasted State
- Starts 12 hours after your last meal
- Natural fat burning state of your body

Fasted state

When the body is in a fasted state, it has several ways to produce energy. Glucose is the body's default fuel, which comes from the carb and sugar-rich foods and stored as glycogen. The liver can deposit around 100 to 150 grams and our muscles about 300 to 500 grams. Within the first 18 to 24 hours of fast, liver glycogen stores are depleted. This significantly decreases blood sugar and insulin levels.

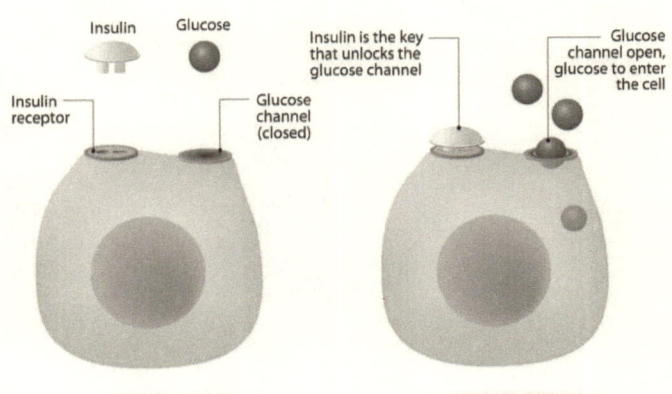

How does insulin work?

The presence of rising blood sugar triggers the insulin release from the pancreas. This happens after you eat your every meal. Insulin's job is to carry them to the body cells for energy and store the excess as fat. The opposite of insulin is glucagon and pancreases also produce it. Glycogen is released when glucose is low. Liver than stats to convert stored glycogen into glucose. The initial phase of fasting is characterized by a high-rate creation of new glucose (gluconeogenesis) with the use of amino acids from bones and muscles.

As fasting continues, the liver starts to produce ketone bodies, which are derived from our own fat cells. Breakdown of stored triglycerides in the adipose tissue (lipolysis) and ketogenesis increase significantly due to fatty acid mobilization and oxidation.

Fasting induces ketosis very rapidly and puts the body into its more efficient metabolic state. The more keto-adapted you become the more ketones you will successfully produce. Keto-adaptation cannot occur in the presence of excess carbohydrates. So, ideally, you should follow the Ketogenic diet when fasting. This will guarantee weight loss.

Chapter 3: Why Fast?

In this chapter, we are going to discuss your reasons for intermittent fasting.

Eating three main meals every day requires a substantial effort from your digestive system because it needs to process, digest and absorb food that you eat non-stop. For many of us, our appetite-regulating brain centers are not strong enough to effectively monitor our daily food intake. Through evolution, our bodies have developed various protective mechanisms to avoid nutritional deficiencies and starvation. But in modern times, food is readily available, and this protective mechanism of our body has become redundant. This has created a problem for us, and this is why obesity is a big health problem today. Let's discuss the health benefits of intermittent fasting:

1. Promotes weight loss: Developing an eating habit that includes regular fasting provides you with many health benefits, including weight loss. At the initial stage of your fast, your body will be forced to burn body fat to produce energy. When you fast, your insulin production is low and your body can access fatty tissues and burn them for energy. Burning body fat to generate energy instead of consumed food will help you to shed excess body fat and also prevent a future fat cell buildup. Fasting will make you look attractive, and you will feel healthier than ever before.

Intermittent fasting can increase the production of one important fat-burning hormones in your body – human growth hormone (HGH). HGH helps break up stored fat cells in your body and plays a crucial role when it comes to losing weight. Here, six studies show the connection between fasting and HGH, the benefits and last three show how IF triggers weight loss:

- https://www.ncbi.nlm.nih.gov/pmc/articles/PMC4590220/
- https://www.ncbi.nlm.nih.gov/pubmed/1548337
- https://www.ncbi.nlm.nih.gov/pubmed/10751442
- https://www.ncbi.nlm.nih.gov/pubmed/16432628
- https://www.ncbi.nlm.nih.gov/pmc/articles/PMC329619/
- https://www.ncbi.nlm.nih.gov/pubmed/2355952
- https://www.sciencedirect.com/science/article/pii/S193152441400200X
- https://www.sciencedirect.com/science/article/pii/S0303720715300800?via%3Dihub
- https://jamanetwork.com/journals/jamainternalmedicine/fullarticle/2623528?utm_campaign=articlePDF&utm_medium=articlePDFlink&utm_source=articlePDF&utm_content=jamainternmed.2017.0936

2. Reduces inflammation: Studies show that intermittent fasting significantly reduces inflammation. It is the inflammation that triggers weight gain and dangerous belly fat. Many modern diseases, including obesity, diabetes, heart disease, dementia, and Alzheimer's are triggered by inflammation.

- https://www.ncbi.nlm.nih.gov/pubmed/21527899

- https://www.ncbi.nlm.nih.gov/pubmed/17291990/
- https://www.ncbi.nlm.nih.gov/pubmed/17374948
- https://www.sciencedaily.com/releases/2017/02/170223124259.htm

3. Boost metabolism: Your body's metabolism increases during short-term food deprivation. This result in a steady weight loss provided that, dieter does not eat or drink excessive carb and sugar-rich food on non-fasting times or days.

- https://www.sciencedirect.com/science/article/pii/S0104423013000213

4. Controls appetite: Intermittent fasting reduces if not completely eliminate your food craving. Since the beginning of the creation, fasting is helping us by acting as a protective mechanism against malnutrition and hunger. Human appetite is not a useful tool to control or manage food intake because it always craves for more food even if our body doesn't need it. The part of the brain that helps control our food craving is located in our lower brain centers and not controlled by higher brain parts responsible for common logic and reasoning. Intermittent fasting trains our bodies to adjust to the short-term absence of food and use the available food more efficiently without storing excess fat in the body.

5. Lowers blood sugar, steady insulin levels, and reverse diabetes: The beneficial effect of intermittent fasting on your blood sugar and insulin production is just as great as weight loss and probably even more important. Short-term food deprivation results in more effective use of blood sugar and improves the use of insulin by your cells. Steady insulin levels without any spikes are the key to losing extra body fat and keeping it off from your body permanently.

   Intermittent fasting helps to lower your blood sugar level and increase your body's tissue sensitivity to insulin at the same time. This prevents pre-diabetes symptoms and helps to prevent diabetes. Studies show that overweight and obese people, who are prone to diabetes, benefit from intermittent fasting. Several clinical studies have revealed that following an intermittent diet for only 14 days can help balance insulin levels. Fasting will help your body to continue to stay in a fat-burning state.

- https://www.sciencedirect.com/science/article/pii/S193152441400200X
- https://www.ncbi.nlm.nih.gov/pubmed/17316625
- https://www.ncbi.nlm.nih.gov/pubmed/15833943

6. Lowers cholesterol: Fasting lowers cholesterol levels in your body, which helps prevent high blood pressure and heart disease. Habitual daily non-stop food consumption may be associated with the cholesterol buildup in your small arteries. Studies show people who are overweight and obese have a greater risk of hypertension, low blood circulation, heart attack, heart disease, and stroke. Besides weight loss,

intermittent fasting helps you to lose weight and naturally lowers cholesterol levels at the same time. Fasting will boost your cardiovascular fitness and remove bad cholesterol from your system.

- https://www.sciencedaily.com/releases/2014/06/140614150142.htm
- https://idmprogram.com/fasting-lowers-cholesterol-fasting-16/

7. Beneficial for heart health: Various risk factors such as blood triglycerides, total and LDL cholesterol, and blood pressure increases your risk of heart disease. Intermittent fasting lowers all these risk factors and reduces your risk of heart disease.

- https://www.ncbi.nlm.nih.gov/pubmed/19793855
- https://ibimapublishing.com/articles/ENDO/2014/459119/
- https://www.ncbi.nlm.nih.gov/pmc/articles/PMC5411330/

8. Fasting improves your immune system: Intermittent fasting aid in regulating inflammatory conditions in your body, lowers free-radical damage and fight's cancer cell formation. All these have a positive effect on your immune system. You may have seen on TV, when animals get sick, they stop eating and start to rest/fast. This process is known as the animal primal instinct to lower stress on their internal system so their body can have the energy to fight infection and other problems. Regrettably, humans are the only species that look for food, even when they

have developed a number of food-related health conditions and don't need any excess food.

9. Fasting promotes healing: When you fast, it creates a dynamic "ripple effect" on your body. The general theory is that fasting helps to de-stress dieter's body. According to health studies, 70% of our daily energy is spent on a number of internal bodily functions such as digesting food and detoxification. If you are living a hectically busy life and don't offer your body the best conditions to rest and heal, then sooner or later diseases will catch up with you. The reason is, similar to your home; your body can sometimes become "dusty and dirty" with toxins and waste matter from the food you eat and the environment around you.

   If your body is clean and working perfectly, it can remove toxins and waste matter effectively. However, when your body is overloaded with toxins and waste matter, it can become lethargic and more prone to diseases. Observations on both humans and animals have shown that when the body goes a brief period without food. It removes damaged mitochondria and replaces them with energy-efficient new ones. Additionally, during a fast, the process of removal of the dead and dying body cells is accelerated.

- https://www.ncbi.nlm.nih.gov/pmc/articles/PMC3106288/
- https://www.ncbi.nlm.nih.gov/pubmed/21106691
- https://www.ncbi.nlm.nih.gov/pubmed/19524509
- https://www.ncbi.nlm.nih.gov/pubmed/23773064

10. Improves brain function: Intermittent fasting increases the production of a protein known as a brain-derived neurotrophic factor (BDNF). This protein improves your brain function. This protein aids brain stem cells to transform into new neurons and release other chemicals that promote neural health. The BDNF protein also protects your brain cells from diseases like Alzheimer's and Parkinson's. Fasting can lower your risk of stroke.

- https://www.ncbi.nlm.nih.gov/pmc/articles/PMC151440/
- https://www.ncbi.nlm.nih.gov/pmc/articles/PMC3022308/
- https://www.ncbi.nlm.nih.gov/pubmed/11220789
- https://onlinelibrary.wiley.com/doi/full/10.1046/j.0022-3042.2001.00747.x
- https://www.ncbi.nlm.nih.gov/pubmed/16011467
- https://www.ncbi.nlm.nih.gov/pmc/articles/PMC2844782/
- https://www.ncbi.nlm.nih.gov/pubmed/17306982

11. Intermittent fasting can help you prevent cancer: Various animal studies show that intermittent fasting can help prevent cancer.

- https://www.ncbi.nlm.nih.gov/pubmed/3245934
- https://www.ncbi.nlm.nih.gov/pubmed/22323820

- https://www.ncbi.nlm.nih.gov/pubmed/16126250
- https://www.ncbi.nlm.nih.gov/pubmed/11835290
- https://www.ncbi.nlm.nih.gov/pubmed/20157582/

As you can see, fasting gives you various health benefits.

Risks of fasting

o There are very few risks of fasting for someone who is well-nourished, to begin with. One major risk is "refeeding syndrome,". The refeeding syndrome is a dangerous condition for malnourished person who starts eating again after a long period (10 days or more) of no food intake. You may find them in the parts of Sub-Saharan Africa or some parts of Asia, and it is caused mainly because of poverty. So it is not a risk of people living in the US or Europe. If you like to fast longer, then keep your fasts under five days, and eat a nourishing diet when you are not fasting.

o If you start fasting but don't eat a diet rich in vitamins, minerals, and essential fatty acids, then you will risk your health.

o Fasting can cause dehydration. So drink lots of fluids and replace your electrolytes, especially if you are exercising.

o You may experience some discomfort as a beginner faster. The hunger hormone ghrelin triggers hunger, and it comes and goes in waves. Keep yourself busy to avoid focusing on food.

Safety measures

There are people that shouldn't fast:

o Pregnant and nursing women – the effects on the baby and fetus are currently unknown. So, it is better not to fast if you are pregnant or nursing.

o Children: Children are still growing and they don't need to fast.

o People with certain medical conditions: People who suffer from liver or kidney weakness or disease should avoid fasting.

o People who have anorexia or bulimia shouldn't fast.

o You should not fast before or after surgery.

o Anyone who is afraid of fasting should avoid fasting

Chapter 4: Busting Myths and Misconceptions of Fasting

Here are the myths and misconceptions of fasting:

1. Fasting puts you in "starvation mode": During WWII, a ground of young men gone through a very low-calorie diet for 6 months for the scientific reasons. Since then, the "starvation mode" became a mysterious bogeyman and scare people who missed even a single meal. If a short-term fasting was harmful, then the human race wouldn't have survived. Our hunter-gatherer ancestors survived the long winters with little food in the Paleolithic era. You will not go into a starvation mode with IF.

2. Fasting triggers muscle loss: Another myth is that fasting burns muscle, but it is not true. The human body evolved to survive periods of fasting. We store food energy as body fat and use this as fuel when food is not available. When food is unavailable, your body uses body fat for energy and only burns muscle when body fat is at less than 4%. As an example, super fit male marathon runners carry about 8% body fat. Almost all of us are not that fit and carry more fat, so our body can burn it for energy. Additionally, this study shows doing alternate day fasting for 70 days lower body weight by 6%, fat mass decreased by 11.4 and lean mass (muscle and bone) did not change.

- http://www.beck-shop.de/fachbuch/leseprobe/9783642290558_Excerpt_001.pdf

3. Fasting triggers low blood sugar: Some worry that fasting will cause low blood sugar, and they will become shaky and sweaty. However, this is not the case. The human body

observes blood sugar levels closely and there are several mechanisms in place to keep it in the proper range. When we fast, your body starts to break down the stored glucose in the liver and keeps the blood level steady. Normally, this happens every night when you sleep.

4. You have to eat 5 to 6 small meals: A lot of people get this advice. We are told that eating frequently will keep your metabolism going and prevent your body from entering starvation mode. The logic behind this theory is that eating small meals continually will cause you to burn more fat. However, the fact is the exact opposite of the truth and has never been proven. For you to actually burn fat & lose weight, you should try to widen the fasting window.

5. Fasting causes overeating: Many people recommend never missing a meal because it could make you extra hungry and cause you to overeat. You may feel hungrier when you start fasting as a beginner. However, with repeated fasting, you will notice the opposite effect. Study on hundreds of fasting patients shows that, over time, appetite tends to decrease as fasting duration increases.

6. Fasting deprives the body of nutrients: There are two types of nutrients, micronutrients, and macronutrients. Micronutrients are vitamins and minerals, and macronutrients are carbs, fats, and proteins. Micronutrient deficiency is extremely rare in the developed world. Additionally, you are doing maximum 24-hour fast. Eat nutrient-dense foods to make up for missed meals and micronutrients. Take a general multivitamin for a longer fast. When comes to macronutrients, it can be helpful to follow a low-carb diet, before and after fasting. Fasting is not a good option for children, pregnant women, and breastfeeding women.

7. Intermittent fasting is bad for women: This depends on the woman's genetic makeup. Experts say that pre-menopausal women may experience hormonal changes during fasting. However, this is mainly seen during extreme fasting (like 36 hours). The reason why intermittent fasting may not be easy for women is that women are more susceptible to stress and fasting being a body stressor makes some women unable to handle it. There are many women who fast 20 hours regularly without any health problem.

8. Breakfast is the most important meal of the day: When you first wake up in the morning, your insulin level is low, and your body is starting to enter the fasted state. The worst thing you could do is eat a meal. It causes glucose and insulin spike and stops fat burning. A better choice would be to wait for a few hours, so your body can fully enter the fasted state and burn stored body fat. Throughout human evolution, we have always been hunter-gatherers, rather than eating a big breakfast first thing in the morning. We would hunt and gather throughout the day and have a larger meal later in the day. A study compared eating breakfast vs. skipping breakfast in 283 overweight and obese adults. After the 16-week study period, there was no difference in weight between groups. So, breakfast is not as important as you thought. Study:

- https://academic.oup.com/ajcn/article/100/2/507/4576452

9. Your metabolism slows down when you fast: This is also not true. Studies show that during fast; metabolism does not slow down. In fact, it might speed up slightly because of the release of catecholamines (dopamine, norepinephrine, adrenaline or epinephrine) and activation of the sympathetic nervous system. SNS is considered the fight or flight system, the opposite of the parasympathetic nervous system; also known as rest and digest system. It is logical that the sympathetic nervous system or fight or flight system activated during the daytime (when

hunter-gatherer humans ware most active, looking for food and in a fasted state) followed by the parasympathetic nervous system or rest and digest mood in the evening after eating a large meal.

10. Fasting lowers your testosterone levels: This is also false, but a bit more complex. Testosterone levels drop after prolonged fasting but come up and even higher after weeks of fasting. With normal fasting, such as 24-hour fast, can actually increase testosterone levels.

Chapter 5: Choose Your Fasting Plan

Common Intermittent Fasting Schedules

	Time-Restricted Eating	5:2	Alternate-Day Fasting	Time-Restricted Eating Plus A 24 Hour Fast
Mon	Eat only from 12 p.m.–8 p.m.	Eat normally	Eat normally	Eat only from 12 p.m.–8 p.m.
Tue	Eat only from 12 p.m.–8 p.m.	24-hour fast	24-hour fast	Eat only from 12 p.m.–8 p.m.
Wed	Eat only from 12 p.m.–8 p.m.	Eat normally	Eat normally	24-hour fast
Thu	Eat only from 12 p.m.–8 p.m.	24-hour fast	24-hour fast	Eat only from 12 p.m.–8 p.m.
Fri	Eat only from 12 p.m.–8 p.m.	Eat normally	Eat normally	Eat only from 12 p.m.–8 p.m.
Sat	Eat only from 12 p.m.–8 p.m.	Eat normally	24-hour fast	Eat only from 12 p.m.–8 p.m.
Sun	Eat only from 12 p.m.–8 p.m.	Eat normally	Eat normally	Eat only from 12 p.m.–8 p.m.

In this chapter, we are going to discuss different types of intermittent fasting methods.

1. The 16/8 Method: The plan calls for 16 hours of fasting and 8 hours of eating window. The extended 8 to 10 hours of eating window gives you the chance to eat two or even three meals. Fitness expert Martin Berkhan invented this fasting method and known as Leangains protocol. The plan calls for 16 hours fast for men and 14 to 15 hours fast for women. You can follow a simple approach to start fasting with this method – don't eat anything after dinner and skip breakfast the next morning. This will give you about 16 hours of fast without difficulty. You skipped one meal, and in theory, you fasted for 16 hours. However, this plan is difficult for people who love to eat breakfast. You can drink no-calorie beverages such as no sugar added tea or coffee during the fast to subdue hunger. Eat real food after fast to get the optimum health benefits.

- https://www.youtube.com/watch?v=D2DUABz0i70&t=1s

2. Alternate-Day Fasting: This plan calls for fasting one day and then eating, as usual, the next day and repeat. This plan has various options, and some of them allow eating approximately 500 calories during the fasting day to make things easier for

the dieter. A 24-hour full fast might be difficult for you and not recommended for the beginners. This plan is for true fast lovers who are willing to stay hungry several times weekly.

- https://www.youtube.com/watch?v=UUb6jugK-iI

3. The Warrior Diet: A known fitness expert Ori Hofmekler introduced this fasting plan in the general population. With this fasting plan, you eat a small number of fruits and raw vegetables during the day and eat a big dinner at night. With this plan, you fast all day and eat a big meal within the 4-hour eating window. This diet plan is one of the pioneers of intermittent fasting and ideal for a beginner like you. The diet includes real, whole, unprocessed food and similar to the Paleo diet.

- https://www.youtube.com/watch?v=dH5rpN1HIS0&t=1s

4. The 5:2 Diet: With this plan, you eat as usual for 5 days and then take about 500 to 600 calories during the rest of the 2 days. The diet is also known as the Fast Diet and introduced by Michael Mosley. It is suggested that with this plan, men take 600 calories and women take 500 calories.

- https://www.youtube.com/watch?v=VWtaLLjJzn4&t=3s

5. Eat-Stop-Eat: With this plan, you fast full 24-hours one or two days of the week. Fitness expert Brad Pilon invented this method and popular among dieters. To perform this fast, you can start fast from Saturday night dinner to Sunday night dinner, and you have done a full 24-hour fast! You can also try breakfast-to-breakfast or lunch-to-lunch method. You can drink water, tea, coffee and or no-calorie beverages during the fast but no solid food. To lose weight, it is important that you eat normally during your eating window. You can start with 16 hours fast and then gradually increase fasting time.

- https://www.youtube.com/watch?v=z9YKnQEM_ps

6. Fat Loss Forever: Dan Go and John Romaniello introduced this fasting plan. This diet plan takes the best parts of Leangains, the Warrior Diet, Eat-Stop-Eat and combines all in one eating plan. With this plan, you get a cheat day followed by a prolonged 36-hour fast. The rests of the days are divided between several different fasting routines. The plan follows a calendar to make things easier for the faster.

- https://www.youtube.com/watch?v=R9ylS3jpyBE&feature=youtu.be

7. Three-day fast: This fast can be done as often as required: Some people decide to start this diet to know how it goes. If 3 days seem a little overwhelming, opt for 24 or 48 hours. Drink mostly water during this time. Aim to drink between 2 to 3 liters of water daily. This can be great to get yourself acquainted with fasting and know how your body reacts before making a permanent decision.

- https://www.youtube.com/watch?v=lJJiFGvN3ag&feature=youtu.be

8. Spontaneous Meal Skipping: No need to follow a structured fasting plan. Skip meals and fast whenever you want. For example, if you are not hungry for dinner, skip it, then delay your breakfast and eat at midday to complete a fasting plan.

Chapter 6: Get Started as a Beginner

If you never skipped a meal before, then fasting is a new event to you. Don't worry, there are things that you can do to make the transition easier and lower the psychological barrier to fasting.

1. Group your eating moments: First, distinguish mealtimes from all other events. Eat your meals during breakfast, lunch, or dinnertime and remember that all other time is non-eating time. Eat your dessert soon after you finished your dinner. Similarly, don't eat before or after breakfast. If you normally eat a snack before lunch, then a snack after lunch. Then eat nothing until dinner.

2. Drink no-sugar tea or coffee: Many of us drink tea or coffee several times a day. Beverages offer many health benefits, but it is the added sweetener that causes trouble. They become another source of sugar in our daily diet and continue to reinforce the sugar cravings that you are trying to subdue. Learn to take your tea plain and coffee black. Add heavy cream, coconut oil or cinnamon, but don't add milk. Don't add anything that has alternative sweeteners, or carbohydrates.

3. Create a "no eating" buffer before your sleep time: If you are eating three meals a day and not snacking in between, then the next step is to create a "no eating" window after dinner and before breakfast. Sleep is a form of Fast, and you can extend it by avoiding eating anything after dinner. For example, if you eat an early dinner at 7, then avoid eating anything before going to bed and push your breakfast out two hours into the day, then you will fast 12 or more hours without actually following any fasting protocol. Fasting for 12 hours is a real accomplishment for a beginner. Next, you can skip breakfast, and eat only during lunch and fast for 16 hours.

4. Discuss with others: Fear of the unknown is one of the biggest challenges when it comes to fasting. Fasting is not a part of Western society, and this is why it is much more intimidating. Ask around your circles and find out who has a fasting practice, whether for health, weight loss, religious, or other reasons. Join various Facebook and other social media groups and know as much as possible. These days, quite a few people are actually fasting. So, you will find several people among your coworkers, friends, and neighbors are fasting. Find support to get started.

5. **Find a support person who will fast with you:** Try to find a person who will fast with you; it will make fasting easier. It could be your friend, your family member, or your partner or spouse. Preferably, someone you share meals with, so you can organize the fast around your meal schedule and either do something else together during mealtimes or break your fast together if the time is right. Finding a fasting partner creates accountability and companionship. The shared experience will motivate both to continue fasting.

6. Don't eat before you exercise: Don't drink a smoothie or have a snack before a workout. Exercise when you are fasting and drink water. Don't worry, you will be fine. If you are hesitant about skipping the snack, then exercise slowly, but continue to avoid snacking. It is likely that you will feel okay after exercise. However, use common sense. If you are obese, not comfortable with exercising, and never fasted, then don't start a big exercise session in the middle of your fast. Do everything gradually – start a short fast, then an extended fast. Understand how you feel and then start exercising.

7. Avoid thinking "I have to eat." We are raised with people saying how much we "have to" eat at the dinner table. Modern lifestyle and society tell us that we "have to" eat three meals a day and snack twice. Presumably, we eat 5 times a day to

"keep up the energy" or avoid low blood pressure. The reality is that we don't need to eat 5 times a day. Remember, eating 5 to 6 times a day is a choice, not a necessity. Start saying to yourself, "I will eat now because it feels right for this situation, but I don't actually need to eat."

8. Give your meal your full attention: With intermittent fasting, you are not mindlessly nibbling throughout the day, devote your full attention to your meal when you are eating. Now you have overcome the "have to eat" scenario. So, you will feel more empowered when you devote time to eating. Stop whatever you are doing and focus on your meal. Don't work, read, drive while you are eating. If you only have a short time, then use that time to eat mindfully. Sit down to your meal without distraction. You will appreciate the experience more.

9. Lower your sugar consumption: Eating sugar-rich food causes your appetite to swing wildly, which makes it difficult for you to fast without snacking (so essentially you are not fasting). Avoid ice cream, cakes, candies, cookies, and all the sugar-rich drinks. Ideally, you should avoid anything that includes added sugar. Intermittent fasting can be a quite difficult experience for you if you eat these foods on a regular basis. The good news is, once you start to avoid the sugar-rich foods; your sugar cravings will go away rather quickly. First, try seven days of no sweets, or only eat something sweet once per day.

10. Start eating more fat: Eating fats make you feel full quickly, you feel satisfied and go longer between meals. Avoid anything labeled as "low-fat" and chose full-fat products. Eat avocados with your meals, use tahini as a dip or sauce for vegetables and eat nuts.

11. Observe your current eating patterns: This will help you start your fast protocol. Observe for a few days, when you eat, and

what you eat. Maybe you are a heavy breakfast eater, or maybe you eat nothing at all in the morning. Take note of your eating pattern. Use your eating habit to incorporate fasting in your life. For example, if you enjoy eating breakfast, then eat a heavy breakfast and fast the rest of the day, or if you regularly skip breakfast, then avoid eating breakfast and eat during lunchtime. So, you will fast from dinner to next-day lunch. This way, you are using your eating habit and making things easier when fasting.

12. Observe your hunger patterns: One of the biggest challenges in starting a fasting protocol is the fear of being hungry. Remember, you are not always hungry when you reach for food. While you are observing your eating patterns, also notice your hunger patterns. Ask yourself these questions:

- Am I hungry before eating something?

- How soon I feel hungry again after eating a meal?

- Is feeling hungry promotes me to seek out food?

- Am I eating not because I am hungry, but because it is meal time, and I need to eat something?

Start a food diary:

kabrita Nutritional Sciences
Diet Diary

Day	Breakfast	Snack	Lunch	Snack	Dinner	Drinks	Symptom/intensity	Comments
Monday								
Tuesday								
Wednesday								
Thursday								
Friday								
Saturday								
Sunday								

13. Set clear goals: What you want to achieve with fasting? Set clear goals and be specific. The reasons can be "I want to be healthy," or "I want to lose weight" and so on. Set goals that are clear and easy to measure. Your goal should be "SMART." SMART stands for:

- Specific: I want to lose weight

- Measurable: I want to lose 4 pounds of weight

- Achievable: I want to lose 1 pound of weight every week

- Realistic: I will start with 12-hour fast, then move on to 16-hour fast.

- Time-bound: I will lose 4 pounds in one month

14. If you are still not sure: If you are still not sure, then just start. It is easy to start fasting. Skipping breakfast and doing a 12-hour fast is very easy for a beginner. Start today because there is no time like the present.

Chapter 7: Avoiding Common Fasting Mistakes

Intermittent fasting offers many health benefits. However, beginners often fail to attain these benefits because of a few mistakes. Here are some of the common mistakes:

1. Excuse to eating junk foods: Often beginners assume intermittent fasting will act as a silver bullet and solve all the problems. They don't really care about the foods they eat as long as they observe the fasting hours as required. You need to focus on eating whole and healthy foods and not junk foods. If you keep eating junk food, and you also claim to be fasting, then you will find yourself with no valuable results at the end of the set period. Eating junk will only act to derail the process of realizing your desired goal and perfect health.

2. Undereating during the eating window: Once you successfully completed your fast, whether it was 12 hours or 16 hours, ensure that you eat enough food as you would normally eat. Some people tend to undereat during the fasting window that negatively affects their body. Take your time and eat mindfully and ensure that the foods that you are eating are whole, fresh and healthy. Since the body is already in a fasting state, eating low carb foods are great and can help with furthering the process of burning fat for fuel, which leads to improved benefits.

3. Failure to drink enough water: When the body is in a fasted state, it begins to breakdown the damaged components while it also detoxifies the body, and this happens since there is no much focus to digestion of food. The intake of a lot of fluids and water is vital during fasting times because the water helps in flushing out the detoxified waste from the body.

4. Obsessing over eating windows: Unconsciously, most of us are living from meal to meal. Most of the people are so focused on eating and every moment is spent on thinking about the foods they will be eating and how hungry they feel. Many people are afraid of being hungry and have the habit of eating something as soon as they begin to sense some feeling of hunger. There are also those who are so conscious of their muscle mass that they eat something as soon as they feel hungry. Fasting helps you to identify true hunger and false craving. You will notice 12, 16 or even 24 fast is completely safe for you.

5. Fasting for many days per week: Fasting can be done at least for 2 to 4 days and anything more than that can be quite exhausting. Fasting for many days within a week can also impact your body performance, metabolism, and appetite. This over fasting can cause hormonal imbalance, especially in women. Don't get obsessed with fasting. Moderation is the key.

6. Intense training while fasting: Another mistake is engaging in intense training during fast. Intense training for a long period of time during fasting can have negative consequences. Exercise, but don't overdo it.

7. Avoid other stressors: Intermittent fasting can be intense for beginners. Adding other stressors can only make the situation to be quite intense, as it requires more energy from you.

Chapter 8: Intermittent Fasting and the Ketogenic Diet

The Ketogenic diet and fasting

On a Ketogenic diet, your macronutrient ratios will be 65 to 70% fat, 15 to 20% protein, and 5 to 10% carbs. The two biggest mistakes' people make when following a Ketogenic diet are eating too many vegetables and not eating enough fat. Remember, you can't eat an unlimited amount of vegetables because they have carbs! Cucumbers, broccoli, and kale, all have carbs. They offer a small number of carbs, but if you eat a large amount of vegetables than you will consume more carbs than the diet recommends. You also can't eat a lot of protein. You can't eat four chicken thighs or a 10-ounce steak at every meal. Over consuming more protein interferes with ketosis.

Here are the benefits you will get if you combine intermittent fasting with Ketogenic diet:

1. Entering ketosis sooner: The Ketogenic diet promotes your body to run on ketones. Ketones are generated when your body starts to use fat for fuel because you are consuming a limited amount of carb. With intermittent fasting, you are already "fasting" yourself from carbs and glucose. With Ketogenic, your aim is reaching ketosis, and intermittent fasting can help you get into ketosis sooner. At the same time, the Ketogenic diet makes IF more tolerable because your body is already adapted to fasting with ketones. Additionally, fat rich keto meals keep you fuller for longer. So, you can fast for an extended amount of time.

2. Avoiding ketosis side effects: Combining IF and Keto can help you avoid a common side effect keto flu. Fat cell shrinkage and switching to ketones triggers the keto flu. Additionally,

combine keto diet with IF makes your fasting more tolerable. If you are eating a carb-rich diet and fasting, your body is constantly switching to glucose when you eat and to ketones when you fast. When you eat a keto diet and fast, your body don't have to switch. It can keep running on ketones.

3. Losing weight faster: One of the biggest reasons people follow the Ketogenic diet is because of weight loss. However, if you follow only keto diet, then it is difficult to overcome weight loss plateaus. Here is how IF helps you with weight loss plateaus:

o IF allows you to limit your calorie consumption.

o Limited eating window helps you avoid snacking.

o IF and keto diet jointly reduces appetite and increase satiety levels.

This study shows that the combination can help you burn more fat:

o https://www.ncbi.nlm.nih.gov/pmc/articles/PMC5064803/

4. Stabilizing blood sugar: Eating a carb-rich diet and fasting force your body to alternate between glucose and ketones for energy. This causes mood swings, brain fog, blood sugar spike, low energy, and other side effects. Combining IF and keto helps you stay in ketosis even when you eat.

Chapter 9: Intermittent Fasting for Women

Intermittent fasting's impact on women is a little different from men. Female's reproductive system and metabolism are deeply entwined. Usually, women consume less protein than men and fasting women will obviously consume even less. Consuming fewer protein results in fewer amino acids present in the female body. Amino acids are required to stimulate estrogen receptors and synthesize IGF -1 (insulin-like growth factor in the liver).

IGF -1 assists the progression of the reproductive cycle. So a diet low in protein can lower fertility and sex drive in women. Furthermore, for women, estrogen isn't only needed for reproduction. Women's have estrogen receptors throughout their bodies, including bones and brains. Change in estrogen balance in a woman's body can disrupt metabolic function and result in indigestion problem, mood swing, sluggish bone formation, etc.

Stressors and hormone balance

Hormone imbalance in women can trigger by stressors other than how much food they eat. Few examples of stressors that can imbalance hormone productions:

o Too little rest and recovery

o Too much stress

o Too much exercise

o Illness, infection and chronic inflammation

o Poor nutrition

o Too little food consumption

You can see, not only too little food but also other factors can also cause a hormone imbalance in a female body.

So as a woman what should you do when it comes to Intermittent fasting?

Now you know that prolong periods of lack of food is a significant stressor for women body and affect their reproductive health. Good news for you is that the intermittent fasting protocols vary, some more extreme than others like 36 hours fasting, which is also difficult and challenging for healthy males. When fasting, the length of time you fast, your age, nutritional status, exercise and other stresses in your life is relevant.

If you want to do intermittent fasting, then follow a conservative approach. For example, start your fasting after dinner and don't eat for 12 -14 hours. So you will fast from dinner to next-day lunch. With this method, you are basically skipping only one meal –breakfast. Repeat the procedure every alternate day. So 12-14 hours fast followed by a 1-day break and then fast for 12-14 hours again. Obviously, sleeping time will make fasting easier for you. Don't practice any hard workouts during your fasting day and limit yourself to practicing yoga or short HIIT session. Follow a routine that makes sense, suits you and one that you can actually maintain. Eat more protein and fat rich foods when fasting and you will be fine.

Stop Intermittent Fasting if:

o Your notice mood swings

o You always seem to feel cold

o Your digestion slows down noticeably

- You start to develop acne or dry skin
- You have problems falling asleep or staying asleep
- Your menstrual cycle stops or suddenly becomes irregular
- Your heart rate becomes abnormal
- You feel a decline in sex drive
- Your hair falls out
- Your stress tolerance declines
- You recover slowly from injury

Avoid fasting if you have these conditions:
- You are completely new to diet and exercise
- You have a history of an eating disorder
- You don't sleep well
- You are chronically stressed
- If you are pregnant

Chapter 10: Fasting Tips to Make the Fast Work for You

In this chapter, we are going to discuss tips, and tricks to make your fast a success.

1. Know your weight, BMI, and your waist size before starting fasting protocol: These are simple things, but important. There are several websites available that will help you calculate BMI. Measuring your weight and waist size will help you know where you were and where you want to go. Weigh yourself regularly but not obsessively. Once every week is enough.

PROGRESS CHART						
Date	Weight	L/R Arm	L/R Leg	Chest	Waist	Hip

INTERMITTENT FASTING BENEFITS

- Absence of hunger and sugar cravings
- Improved heart health
- Increased brain function
- Chronic disease prevention
- Protects against alzheimers
- Increased life span
- Increased insulin sensitivity
- Increased mitochondrial energy efficiency
- Decreased oxidative stress
- Increased capacity to resist stress, disease, & aging
- Weight Loss

My Personal Intermittent Fasting Benefits:

2. Chart your progress: Have a target in your mind and monitor your progress. Make a realistic plan and write it down. Plenty of people recommend keeping a diet diary. Data shows that dieters who write daily notes are known to be more successful at losing weight than those who don't. (https://www.ajpmonline.org/article/S0749-3797(08)00374-7/abstract).

3. Prep your fast-day food in advance: This approach will help you avoid eating carb and sugar-rich food. Keep it simple, and aim for flavor without effort. Before you start your fast, clear the house of junk food.

4. Breaking your fast: Break your fast gently. The longer the fasting period, the gentler you must be. Often we overeat as soon as the fast is over. Not because of overwhelming hunger, but more of a psychological need to eat. Break your fast with a snack or small dish to start. Then wait 30 to 60 minutes before eating your main meal. This will usually give time for any waves of hunger to pass and allow you to gradually adjust to eating again. Short-duration fasts (such as 24 hours or less) require no special precautions. However, you need to plan ahead for a longer fast. On fast days, eat with awareness, allowing yourself to fully absorb the fact that you are eating. Eat until you are satisfied, not until you are full. Find out what the concept of "fullness" means for you. Here are some suggestions for the first snack:

    o A small amount of meat (two slices of pork belly or three slices of prosciutto)

    o A small bowl of soup

    o A small bowl of raw vegetables with olive oil dressing

- o A small salad
- o A tbsp. peanut butter or almond butter
- o 1/3 cup almonds, walnuts, or macadamia nuts

5. Stay busy: Fill your day to avoid filling your face. Engage in things other than food, anything that appeals to you.

6. Experiment: You need to experiment a little until you find the fasting plan that works for you. Remember, fasting is not a diet, instead; it is "diaita" meaning "manner of living." Experiment and customize your fasting plan.

7. Don't try to suppress the thought of food during fast: A psychological mechanism known as habituation. It means the more people have of something, the less value they attach to it. Meaning trying to suppress the thought of food during fasting is a wrong strategy. See food as a friend, not a foe. Remember, food is not dangerous, supernatural, or magical. Don't demonize it, see it as only food. Don't try to associate fasting with discomfort. If you had to break a fast, then move on. Don't dwell on it.

8. Stay hydrated: Drink plenty of calorie drinks. A dry mouth is the last sign of dehydration, not the first, so act before your body complains. Drink around 8 big glasses of water and/or herbal tea/coffee daily during your fast. Drinking water will also stop you from mistaking thirst from hunger.

9. Exercise caution: Be sensible. If fasting feels uncomfortable to you, then stop. If you are concerned about an aspect of intermittent fasting, see your doctor. Remember, you can break your fast at any time.

10. Congratulate yourself: Every competed fast day is a success for you. The study shows that positive feedback on new habits

will increase the likelihood of success. Don't be afraid of grandstand your fasting achievements.

- https://onlinelibrary.wiley.com/doi/abs/10.1111/j.1751-9004.2010.00285.x

Common Concerns:

Hunger

This is the number-one concern for a beginner faster. People think that when they start fast, hunger will overwhelm them, and they will not be able to control themselves during the fast. Without a doubt, the hunger issue is the most common worry about fasting. Most people worry that they will simply be unable to continue fasting because of hunger. However, researches on fasters reveal that with an intermittent fasting plan, hunger actually diminishes, not increases.

Fasters reveal that they are eating less than half their usual amount of food on a daily basis, yet feel completely full. This is one of the most pleasant surprises of fasting. Usually, we start to feel hunger pangs about four hours after our last meals. So we think that fasting 24-hour creates hunger sensations six times stronger. However, it is not the case. During longer fasts, many people notice that their hunger completely disappears by the second or third day.

Here are some drinks and spices that are allowed on fasts that can help suppress hunger.

o Water: Staying hydrated helps prevent hunger. Sparkling mineral water may help for noisy stomach and cramping.

- Green tea: Antioxidant and polyphenols rich green tea is a great aid for the dieters. Antioxidants help stimulate metabolism and weight loss.

- Cinnamon: Cinnamon slow gastric emptying and helps suppress hunger. It also aids in weight loss.

- Coffee: Both decaffeinated, and regular coffee suppresses hunger better than caffeine in water.

- Chia seeds: Chia seeds are high in soluble fiber and omega-3 fatty acids. These seeds help suppress hunger.

Dizziness

You may experience dizziness because of dehydration. Fasting doesn't cause dizziness. You need to consume both salt and water to cure dizziness. Drink bone broth daily. Also, low blood pressure can cause dizziness, especially if you are taking medications for hypertension. Speak to your physician about adjusting your medication.

Headaches

Headaches are common the first few times you fast. Usually, it happens because of the transition from a relatively high-salt diet to the very low salt intake on fasting days. Headaches are temporary and often resolve themselves. Take some extra salt in the form of broth or mineral water.

Constipation

Bowel movements will usually decrease during a fast because there is less food intake. If you are not experiencing any discomfort, then there is nothing to worry about. However, increase your intake of vegetables, fiber, and fruits during the non-fasting days to prevent constipation. Take Metamucil during or after fasting to increase fiber and stool bulk.

Heartburn

Avoid taking large meat after finishing your fast to prevent heartburn. Also, try to stay in an upfront position for at least 30 minutes after meals. Similarly, placing wooden blocks under the head of your bed to raise it may help with nighttime symptoms. Drinking sparkling water with lemon often helps. If the problem continues, consult with your physician.

Muscle Cramps

Low magnesium may cause muscle cramps. You may need an over-the-counter magnesium supplement. You may also soak in Epsom salts, which are magnesium salts. Alternatively, you may apply magnesium oil on your skin.

Chapter 11: Q & A

Which days should I choose to fast?

It is your life, and you will know which days will suit you best. For most of us, Monday is an obvious choice because it is more manageable, both practically, and psychologically. You might want to avoid Saturdays and Sundays. The weekend schedule is full of family lunches, brunches, and dinner dates. So, it is not realistic to fast on the weekend. Thursday is a sensible second fasting day.

When should I eat?

Some fasters appreciate the convenience and simplicity of a single 500/600 calorie evening meal. Some people say they feel hungrier during the day if they have breakfast. Others prefer to eat breakfast and then avoid food for a fasting window of around twelve hours until supper. Remember, over time, you will get used to the intermittent fasting eating pattern as your body gets acclimated to periods of fasting. Stay alert and tweak the regime to suit your needs.

Do I have to go for a 24-hour fast?

Fasting for a day is practical, coherent, and unambiguous. A fast day with its 500/600 calorie allowance lasts up to 36 hours. For example, if you finish your Sunday night dinner at 7:30 pm and Monday is your fast day, you will eat normally again on Tuesday at 7:30 am. So, it is 36 hours.

Fasting on consecutive days

If you do back-to-back fasts, your body will spend longer in the fasted state. Usually, this is a good thing. Many people fast on Monday and Tuesday. However, fasting for two days in a row can make you bored, resentful and beleaguered.

How much weight will I lose?

This will depend on your level of activity, your starting weight, your body type, your metabolism, and how honestly you fast and how much you eat and drink on your non-fast days.

What can I do if I am not losing weight?

- o Be patient. Some people will take longer than others to start losing weight.

- o Be realistic. Losing 1 or 2 pounds per week is normal.

- o Watch what you are eating on your non-fast days. Stay aware and be sensible. Avoid binging.

- o Keep a diary of everything you eat and drink for a week. Then look at the calorie content. Some foods may leap out. Avoid low-fat products.

- o If you are not following keto, then look at the calories you are getting from smoothies, fizzy drinks, alcohol, lattes, and juices.

- o Moving more will certainly help.

- o Try adding another fast day. You can go for 4:3 pattern. Four days of eating and 3 days of fast.

o

Will my blood sugar fall? Will I faint?

Your body evolved to cope with periods without food. There is no evidence that intermittent fasting will cause you to faint. If you are healthy, then your body will effectively manage your blood sugar. Your blood sugar will not drop abnormally during fast, and you will not faint. If you are diabetic, then consult with your doctor.

Will IF lead to muscle breakdown?

Some people fear that intermittent fasting could lead to protein deficiency and muscle breakdown. It is true that once you fast for more than 24 hours, your body will seek amino acids from existing muscle. However, if your protein intake is adequate, then you are not going to get "muscle protein breakdown." Studies show that intermittent fasting can help dieters preserve muscle when compared with a standard diet.

What about alcohol?

Alcoholic drinks merely provide empty calories. Drinking alcohol causes dryness and if you are fasting, the feeling of dryness can make you uncomfortable. So, avoid or limit your alcohol consumption.

Should I take supplements?

Intermittent fasting is an eating pattern, not a deprivation regimen. So, if you eat a healthy, balanced diet, you should get all the vitamins and minerals you require. You don't need any supplements, but if you are fond of them, then you can take these:

o Glucosamine – ideal for relieving joint pain

o Casein Protein – ideal for pre-bedtime

- Whey Protein – Protein boost for pre and post workout
- Beta Alanine – boosts exercise performance
- Creatine – helps boost muscle when working out.
- Branched Chain Amino Acids (BCAA) – can help limit lean body-mass loss as well as increasing visceral fat loss
- Vitamin D – helps you function optimally
- Calcium – increases fast excretion and boosts testosterone.
- Fish oil – helps keep your Omega – 3 and 6 levels up
- Multivitamin – to overcome deficiencies

You will find all the products on Amazon.

Should I exercise on a fast day?

Yes, you can exercise during fast days. Research has shown that even a more extreme three-day fast has no negative effect on the ability to perform, long-duration, moderate-intensity workouts, or short-term, high-intensity exercise. The first study reveals there is no adverse effect when people exercise while fasting. Additionally, exercising while fasting can result in better metabolic adaptations. The last study shows that exercising before breakfast is beneficial for metabolic performance and weight loss.

- https://www.ncbi.nlm.nih.gov/pubmed/19085449
- https://www.ncbi.nlm.nih.gov/pubmed/21051570
- https://www.ncbi.nlm.nih.gov/pubmed/20837645

Let's discuss a bit more on fasting and exercising

The smart way to exercise when fasting:

You don't have to start a vigorous exercising routine if you are maintaining an intermittent fasting plan, but practicing a regular exercise is important for your mental and physical health. Follow these guidelines to get the most out of your fasting:

o Practice low-intensity cardio when fasting: Your breathing is a good indication of the intensity of your exercise. Practicing low-intensity cardio means you should be able to carry on a normal conversation relatively easily while you are exercising. Listen to your body, and if you feel dizzy or light-headed, stop exercising.

o Practice high-intensity after you have broken your fast: If you are practicing intermittent fasting, then HIIT or high-intensity interval training is best for you. These workouts involve walking, running, cycling, swimming and various group exercises - practiced at 80 to 95% of a person's projected maximal heart rate. A few intermittent fasting programs have guidelines about exercising while fasting to maximize fat loss. Usually, you should do high-intensity exercises after you have broken fast and eaten. That way, you will have some surplus ketosis to generate energy for your exercise, and you will avoid the risk of low blood sugar levels.

o Focus on high-protein meals: You should eat before and after exercise if building muscle is your aim. Protein-rich foods will provide amino acids to your muscles to repair and grow. When fasting, the timing of the exercise is important. Exercises like strength training should be between 2 proteins rich meals.

Starting your HIIT exercise

Intensity is the key when practicing HIIT. Ideally, you want your heart rate to elevate to your anaerobic threshold. You can use different intervals of exertion and recuperation. Following is a usual HIIT exercise plan with an elliptical machine:

1. Warm up your body for 3 minutes.

2. Exercise hard and fast for 30 seconds. Exercise should make you feel out of breath and unable to practice for additional few more seconds. Use lower resistance and higher repetitions to steadily increase the heart rate.

3. Recuperate for about 90 seconds, continue to move your body, but at a much slower pace and reduced resistance.

4. Repeat the HIIT and recovery for a few more times.

Depending on your fitness, you may only be able to do 2 or 3 repetitions of HIIT when first starting out. Aim for 20-minute sessions once your body gets fitter.

Gender differences

Fasting benefits both sexes and healthy women can fast without worrying about anything. However, fasting is not meant to be a struggle. If for whatever reason, short bouts of fasting interrupt your menstrual cycle, or your sleep pattern, then modify your approach till you find a comfortable balance that works for you.

Fasting during period

Some women may find fasting more challenging on the days preceding a period. There are no clear studies on the impact of intermittent fasting on the menstrual cycle. So, you can avoid fasting during your period.

Can I fast if I am trying to get pregnant?

There are not enough studies to assess the overall effects of fasting on fertility. Extreme fasting affects fertility in animals, but it also reverses. Err on the side of caution and don't fast when you are trying to get pregnant.

Will go to bed hungry?

It depends on your metabolism and how you timed your fast day calorie consumption. If you feel hungry, take your mind off it – read a good book, take a bubble bath, do a stretch, or drink a cup of herbal tea.

Will hunger affect my sleep?

Some people find it hard to sleep on an empty stomach. So you can drink a glass of milk or a small snack before bed.

Is it too late to start?

On the contrary, there is no time like the present. Intermittent fasting is likely to prolong your life. You will subdue your appetite and lose weight. Fasting will lead to a healthier, leaner, longer old age with fewer doctors' visits.

Chapter 12: Success Stories with Intermittent Fasting

Here are a few weight loss success stories with intermittent fasting:

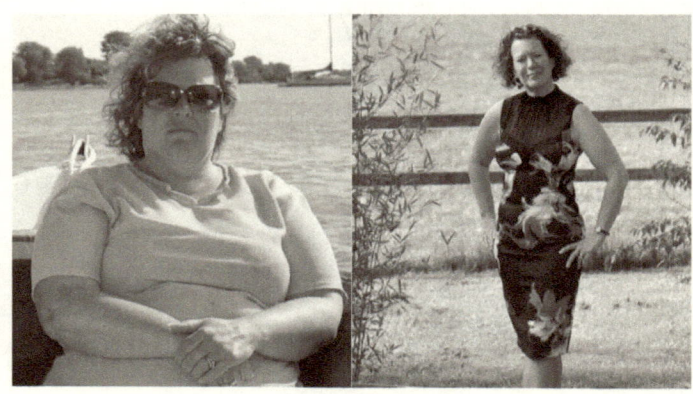

https://www.fastday.com/success-stories/carolines-story/

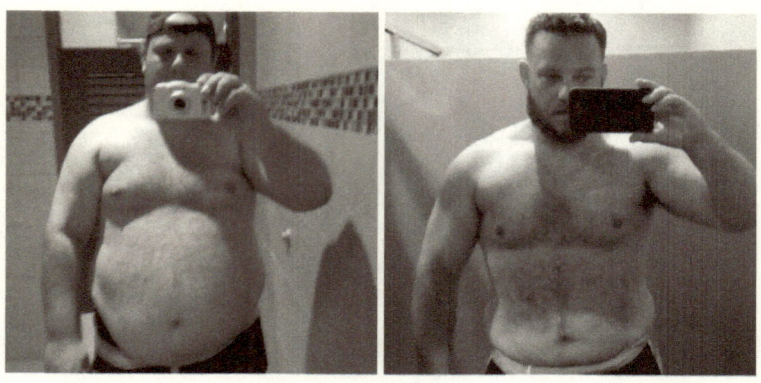

https://beachbaby.net/intermittent-fasting-success-story-interview-james-wanderlust-estate/

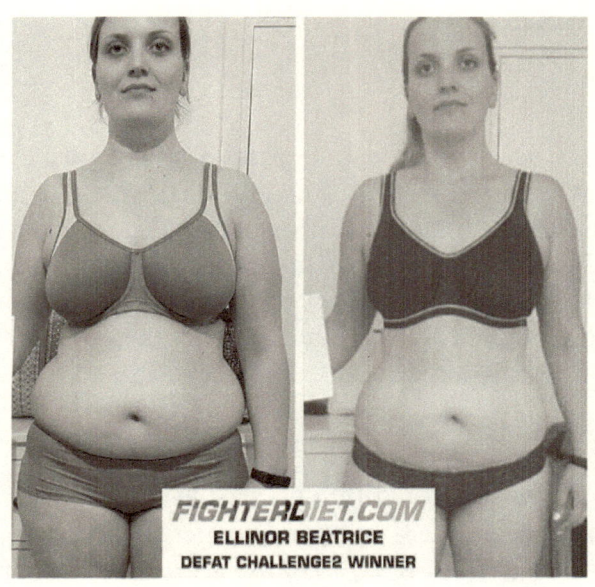

https://fighterdiet.com/success-stories

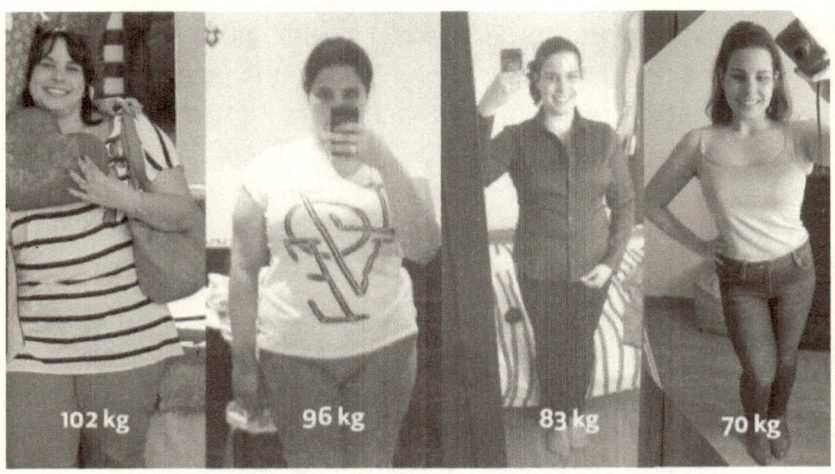

https://www.fastday.com/success-stories/ana-sofias-story/

Conclusion

Intermittent Fasting is an eating pattern where you cycle between periods of eating and fasting, and along with it comes incredible health benefits. It has been proven to reduce weight for the millions who have tried it. The great thing about Intermittent Fasting is that you are not missing out on birthday celebrations, dinner with friends, wedding cakes, and holiday favorites. You can start today without any hassle and feel the benefits soon!

We all want to lose weight for different reasons. It may be for health reasons, to look and feel better or to get in shape for a vacation or an event. The truth is, most of us fail to lose weight or gain weight back within a short period of time. However, Intermittent Fasting is different than your usual diet; it is a lifestyle adjustment toward greater health and wellness. Based on the latest scientific research, this comprehensive guide to Intermittent Fasting will give you all the tips, tricks, and lessons for an easy and permanent weight loss. There is no need to wait. With this complete Intermittent Fasting guide, you will never need another book on the subject.

If you APPLY this you will...

- Reach your *ideal weight* by combining intermittent fasting and ketogenic diet

- *Burn* your useless reserves of *fat* with mathematical methods of fasting-rest-nourishment

- You will know how your body works to take advantage of the processes to your advantage even *while you sleep*

- *Tips* and *tricks* to transform your mentality and live in peace with your body

- become *healthier*, *slim*, *fit* and feel more *energetic*

I hope you enjoyed this eBook. If you learned a few things and found it interesting, I would be very grateful if you would consider leaving me a review with a few kind words.

Thank you very much,

Best wishes from **Self-Publishing Mastery**!

www.ingramcontent.com/pod-product-compliance
Lightning Source LLC
Chambersburg PA
CBHW030524220526
45463CB00007B/2702